Dr. Linzman's Weight Control for Life

Dr. Linzman's Weight Control for Life

This is not a Diet Book

Finally the Truth

Rod Linzman

To order additional copies of this book, contact:
Xlibris Corporation
1-888-795-4274
www.Xlibris.com
Orders@Xlibris.com
51126

CONTENTS

Intro

This book explains how to control your weight for the rest of your life.

It is very simple because that is all most of us will do, including me. You will probably have many questions, but if you will just go back each time to the three rules and three exceptions, they will answer your questions. If I started trying to answer all the "possibilities," this book would be ten times as long and as voluminous. Instead I have chosen to write a short practical and interactive book that is the only truth out there about weight control for life.

The three rules and three exceptions will answer any questions; don't try to make it more complicated than what I have written.

I know this plan will be beneficial to anyone who reads it. To many, it will be life changing, and the idea of having helped someone makes me happy.

Chapter I

CALORIES = WEIGHT

This short chapter may seem a little boring, but it is very important. At least it is short. When we eat or drink things, we take calories into our bodies.

A *calorie* is a measurement of energy. Webster defines it as the amount of heat required to raise one gram of water one degree centigrade. Just think of it as energy.

Our weight is determined by the amount of calories we take in *minus* the amount we burn up by our activity.

Unless you are an extremely active person like a lumberjack, football player, or marathon runner *your weight is mainly* (probably 90 percent) *controlled by what you eat and drink.* In other words—what is crossing your *lips.*

I will have a chapter on exercise, but I want you to understand that, for most of us, 90 percent of what we weigh is controlled by the calories crossing into our body through our mouth.

For an analogy, think of a calorie as a drop of gasoline. If you drink a Coke that has 120 calories, you just put 120 drops of gasoline in your tank. If you walk for thirty minutes, you burn up 120 calories, which means you took 120 drops of gasoline out of your tank.

Weight is simply:

calories in (-) calories out

All the calories that cross your lips minus (-) all the calories you burn up in your daily activities.

Let's pretend your car has a 300-gallon gas tank. Let's also say it has 150 gallons in it now. Next let's say you put 10 gallons of gas in your car everyday so that on day one you start with 160 gallons in your car. Then let's say you burn up 9.9 gallons of gas driving back and forth to work. At the end of day one, you now have 150.1 gallons of gas in your car. Continuing on in this manner, your car will have 300 gallons in it four years, one month, and ten days later.

A more practical analogy is that if you put an extra one hundred calories per day (less than the calories in one Coke) in your body for four years, you will gain forty pounds.

See what I mean? It's a small amount of calories over a long period of time that determines our weight.

CALORIES = WEIGHT!

ALL

CALORIES

COME

INTO

YOUR

BODY

BY

ONE

OF

THREE

WAYS

(Please read out loud.)

1. WHAT YOU *DRINK*

2. WHAT YOU EAT *AT* MEALS

3. WHAT YOU EAT *BETWEEN* MEALS

(Please read out loud.)

Chapter II

HABITS

This is not a diet book. This book explains how to control your weight for the rest of your life.

Diets do not work because they are by definition a plan to *decrease your calories for a certain period of time.*

On a diet, after you have lost the weight you set as your goal or you get tired of the diet, you go back to your old eating habits and you regain the weight.

In other words, if you were taking too many calories in before a diet and return to your old eating habits, then you are returning to taking in too many calories and will gain weight.

14

My plan is *very simple* and it is based on you *changing your eating habits* for the *rest of your life.*

You really do want to change, or you wouldn't be reading this book. The idea of changing for the rest of your life may sound scary at first, but at least hear me out.

First, it is the *only* thing that *works*!

Second, habits *once formed* are *easy* whether they are *good* or *bad.*

We are creatures of habits whether they are good or bad. So why not change to *good* habits?

Again, this book is simple and straightforward with the truth. You have to decide if changing is worth it to you.

The changes I am talking about are only three. I will list them here and then expand on them in three sections. They are:

1. *No*-calorie drinks

2. *One* helping of *any* food at meals

3. What to do *between meals* if you get hungry

That's it! Three rules!

(Please read the three rules above out loud.)

I will expand on them in the next three sections.

Chapter III

RULE NUMBER 1

NO-CALORIE DRINKS

To show you why this is important, let's see what happens when you drink one cola (Coke) that is approximately 120 calories.

1 Coke/day x 30 days = 3,600 calories.

There are 3,500 calories in one pound. Therefore, that is one pound gain in weight in one month.

Twelve months in one year = twelve pounds gain.

If you are thirty-five and you live only to seventy, that is 420 pounds. If you are twenty-five and you live to eighty-five, that is 720 pounds.

These figures don't take into account the calories burned that we would subtract, but I think you can see the picture.

A Coke really has 140 calories. A six-ounce glass of grape juice has 120 calories. A glass of milk has approximately 120 calories.

My example was for only one Coke a day. If you drink a couple of twelve-ounce Cokes and a glass of juice or milk, you can see what happens overtime.

So I'm informing you that if you choose to change your eating habits and adopt rule number 1, you are one-third of the way toward controlling your weight for the *rest of your life*!

I guess the only excuse you can make not to do this is that you like your "favorite drink."

There are so many good drinks available that taste good! To name a few, Diet Dr. Pepper, Diet Pepsi, Diet Root Beer, Fresca, Crystal Light, and on and on. I challenge you to try several, pick one, and drink it for a couple of months, and you will get used to it and enjoy it as much as your present "favorite drink."

How do you do it? Most of my patients take a few days to a few months to get to the point that they like Diet Dr. Pepper, Coke Zero, Crystal Light or some other no-calorie drink.

The thing is that once you change to a new habit, the longer you do it, the easier it becomes.

The change hurts a little for a few months, at the most; but when you get used to it, it is easy.

I would rather drink Diet Dr. Pepper than Dr. Pepper now because I am used to it! It's what you get used to.

The return on your investment of changing from calorie to no-calorie drinks is *great*.

Think about it. One to three months of some suffering in exchange for thirty, forty, or fifty years of benefit payoff, depending on how old you are.

I like the mental picture of drinking a Diet Dr. Pepper and I have two right arms. One arm is drinking Diet Dr. Pepper and the other is throwing calories over my shoulder!

Choice? Suffer some for a month or two versus taking in 1,400,000 or more calories over the next thirty years. (Based on one Coke or milk or juice daily.)

RULE NUMBER 1

NO-CALORIE DRINKS

(Please read out loud)

Chapter IV

RULE NUMBER 2

ONE HELPING AT MEALTIME

Eating is good. You should enjoy it. I want you to commit to eating one helping. Simply put, *no seconds.* If it is mealtime (breakfast, lunch, or dinner) and you are hungry, learn to eat one helping.

How do you do it? Put one helping of food on your plate. (Not as much food as you can get on it—come on, you know what a normal serving is!)

When you get down to the last bite, stand up and eat the last bite.

Then take your plate, walk to the sink, and put it in.

Then immediately *go do something else.*

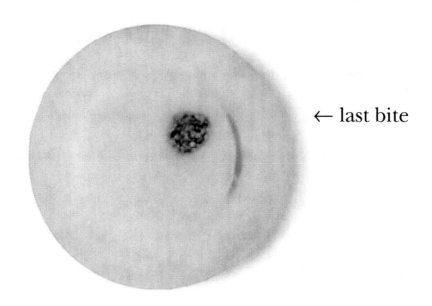

← last bite

The problem with rule number 2 is that a lot of time, you still want to eat after finishing one helping.

What you need to know and learn is that the feeling of hunger after eating one helping goes away in about ten to fifteen minutes *after* you stop eating.

I can eat one chili dog and I'm still hungry. I can eat two chili dogs, and I want another one. Sometimes after three chili dogs, I can still have that feeling of hunger.

But if I stop after one chili dog and do something else (usually a chore around the house or, if at lunch, go back and do some work or go for a walk), I find that one chili dog was enough. Why?

As long as you are eating, your tongue is enjoying the sensation, and your brain doesn't feel satisfied (satiety).

As long as you are eating, the sugar levels and insulin levels are going up.

As long as they are going up, you don't feel satisfied (satiety). As soon as you quit eating and the sugar and insulin levels start dropping, then the brain says it is OK—the feeling of hunger stops. Remember, it only takes ten to fifteen minutes for the sugar levels in your blood to start down, and the desire to eat more goes away.

An example to prove this has been experienced by all of us. Remember sometimes when you were eating dinner and had finished one-half to three-fourths of your meal and the phone rang or the doorbell rang and you spent fifteen minutes visiting? Usually, or a lot of times, your hunger was gone. That was because your sugar and insulin levels dropped, and satiety set in.

You might wonder why I don't say anything about what kind of food. It's because it really isn't about calorie-dense foods.

It's about one helping. Eat pizza, eat fried chicken, potatoes and gravy. *Just eat one helping*!

Think about this. If your one helping has 700 calories and you follow this rule, then you are talking about 2,100 calories a day and that intake will result in maintaining or losing weight.

Think about a meal with only 500 calories and you ate one and a half helpings. You ate 750 calories. If you ate two helpings, that is 1,000 calories.

The difference is 50-250 calories a meal. Let's say you eat more than one helping in two meals a day, that is 100-500 extra calories per day.

We'll split the difference and call it an extra 300 calories a day. Three hundred calories a day for thirty days is 9,000 calories, which is nearly three pounds. Three pounds a month for a year is thirty-six pounds. In ten years, that is three hundred and sixty pounds. You get the point.

So rule number 2: *one helping at meals* really pays off. Remember, once you develop a good habit, it is easy to do.

This rule requires an *action* on your part, *not willpower.* The action is when you get down to the last bite, you stand up and eat that last bite.

Then pick up your plate and put it in the sink.

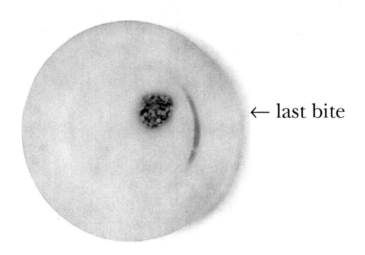

← last bite

When you stand up, you are telling your brain, "I'm almost done." When you put the last bite in your mouth, you are telling yourself, "I'm done."

When you are walking to the sink, you are telling your brain, "I'm done."

When you put your plate in the sink, you are saying again, "I'm done."

Now go do something! In ten to fifteen minutes, the feeling of hunger will go away. Once you establish this habit, it becomes easy—*for the rest of your life*!

It is very important to immediately do something after you put your plate in the sink. <u>Your mind</u> can only do one thing at a time. So instead of suffering with the feeling of hunger, you will have switched your mind to something else and won't "notice" the hunger during that ten to fifteen minutes when your blood sugar levels drop in your blood and brain.

This is a physiological truth that isn't obvious, but nonetheless, it is the way the brain and hunger work. Isn't it *great* to know that hunger, after eating one helping, goes away after ten to fifteen minutes when your blood sugar level drops?

RULE NUMBER 2

ONE HELPING AT MEALTIME

(Please read out loud.)

Chapter V

RULE NUMBER 3

BETWEEN MEALS

I don't know how to pronounce it. It is an acronym for Water, fruit or vegetable, water.

WFOVW

What I'm trying to communicate to you is that if you get hungry and it is between meals, then go as *fast* as you can and drink a glass of water. Eat some fruit or vegetables. Then drink another glass of water.

30

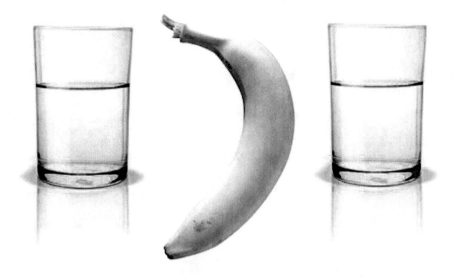

Then ask yourself how you are. "Am I still hungry?" Eighty to ninety percent of the time, that will make the feeling of hunger go away.

If that doesn't satisfy you, then go ahead and eat what you are craving. My wife says that I should tell people to eat some kind of low-calorie snack at this point. I think she is right.

But the important thing is do **WFOVW** as fast as you can. If you get hungry between meals, then don't sit and stew about it—just go for **WFOVW**.

When I say as fast as you can, I mean *starting* the process of **WFOVW**.

I don't mean you have to gulp the water or eat the apple, banana, orange, corn, carrots, celery, green beans, or whatever fruit or vegetable you pick in a hurry—just start the process.

(Since starting this book, they have come out with 100 cal. snack paks and you may substitute this for the fruit or vegetables.)

RULE NUMBER 3

WFOVW

(Please read out loud.)

Water, fruit or vegetable, water

Chapter VI

STRESS AND THE WATCH

Why do we get hungry between meals? Stress. What is stress? I think another word for it is pain.

I don't know anyone who likes pain.

Stress usually comes in a negative form, such as being bored, anxious, worried, mad, or sad. There are positive stresses that also make us hungry—like being happy. How?

Have you ever been watching TV or playing cards and having fun when you noticed it made you feel hungry? I think that is the brain saying, "I want to be *happier.*"

I think we often don't recognize the stress before we find ourselves eating. Why? To relieve the pain (of stress). We have developed a *bad habit* of eating in response to the stress. Usually, this is some kind of high-calorie snack.

So how do you do this WFOVW rule number 3, and how do you do rule number 2 of one helping?

I got an idea!

<u>Look at your watch—anytime you are hungry.</u>

SIMPLE!

Even if you don't wear a watch. I want you to raise your wrist and <u>look</u> at your "watch" whenever you get hungry.

There are only two times on the watch.

1. Mealtime   (rule number 2)
2. Between meals   (rule number 3)

If it is mealtime, then eat one helping of whatever you want.

If it is between meals, then do WFOVW.

I now want you to raise your right hand and take an oath. Please say out loud, "I turn my eating over to my watch."

Now when you are hungry for whatever reason, just <u>look</u> at your watch, and let it <u>tell</u> you what to do. This provides an *action* to engage your *brain* into taking the right action of rules one, two, and three.

Chapter VII

"WHAT'S IN IT FOR ME?"

You can tell me that eating one helping makes you suffer some for ten to fifteen minutes, and I agree, but you can endure this pain by developing the habit. The longer you do it, the easier it gets.

You can tell me it isn't fun to do WFOVW, but it doesn't hurt—it's just not as fun as eating chips or candy or ice cream.

So why should you change your eating habits? Why do you want to be at a certain weight? In other words, "what's in it for me?"

36

People usually do something because there are more benefits in doing it one way or another.

It is *very important* that you fill in the TABLE below so you crystallize in your MIND why you want to change. Feel free to use any of the things I wrote in under EXAMPLES in the right hand column.

Table 1

"So what's in it for me?"

1._____	1. Ex*amples I have thought of*
2._____	2. *Self-esteem*_____
3._____	3. *Clothes* _____
4._____	4. *Health*_____
5._____	5. *Energy*_____
6._____	6. *Feel better*_____
7._____	7. *Breath better*_____
8._____	8. *Save money*_____

You need to fill in the table above. This is what you get out of it! This is what is in it for you. This is why you will benefit from changing to your new rules for living. I think it would be a good idea, after you fill this out, to make a copy of it and put it on your refrigerator or bathroom mirror or in an obvious place you can read every day. You may also just want to tear out the previous page with the table you filled in and place it in an obvious place as mentioned above.

Chapter VIII

"A LITTLE PSYCHOLOGY"

I like to think that there are two people living in all of us, an adult and a child. This child is like a five-year-old the way he/she thinks.

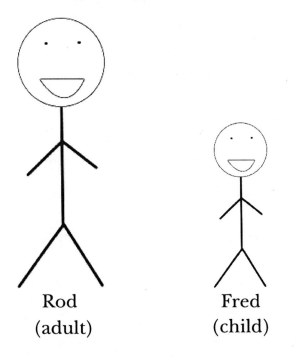

Rod
(adult)

Fred
(child)

Rod (the adult in me) wants all the things in the table I just filled out on page 37. Fred (the child in me) could care less. Fred (the 5 year old child) wants what he wants when he wants it and doesn't care about anything else. When he feels the stress (pain) of life, he wants to eat something to relieve the pain.

Rod (the adult) wants what is in table 1, so he doesn't want to eat extra calories. Fred (the 5 year old child) wants the stress to go away.

So the battle is on!

Fred wants to go to Alaska to fish, but Rod doesn't have the time or money right now.

Fred wants to speed up and get there in a hurry, but Rod doesn't want to pay the ticket.

Fred wants to sleep in, but Rod knows he has to go to work.

Fred wants out of the Navy and so does Rod! So we both got out of the Navy!

So who runs the show?

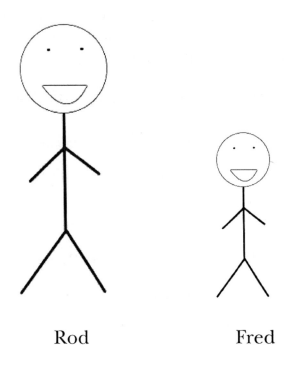

Rod   Fred

Guess what? Rod usually does because the adult really can control the situation. Sometimes we let the child in us control things, but it is *only because we let him or her*! We have given up the power to him or her.

So *you,* the *adult* that is reading this book (the child doesn't even like you reading this), gets to *choose* if you get the things in table 1 or the child gets to make you keep suffering.

You remember me telling you that new rules can become habits? That habits are easy? What I think is going on is that the longer the child in us believes that we are going to follow the three rules then the less he/she complains about them. The child gives up when it finds out we *mean* it.

A child may keep asking to stay up a little longer if we occasionally let them stay up a little longer.

A child quits asking to go play in the traffic because we emphatically say *no*. Then the child says, "Can I play on the edge?"

And we say *no*! Then the child says, "Little Billy gets to play in the traffic." And we say *no*! Then the child says, "I'll be real careful." And we say *no*! The child soon learns that playing in the traffic won't work, so he quits asking.

You get the picture.

So to get the things in table 1, you have to decide to follow the three rules. I don't think they are that hard or unreasonable.

They are based on taking <u>actions</u>:

1. Getting up at the last bite

2. WFOVW

3. No-calorie drinks

I am not asking you to use willpower not to eat. I'm asking you to take *action* and *eat* if you are hungry for whatever cause, just *eat* according to your three new simple rules.

Chapter IX

RED LIGHTS

Red lights are easy to stop at. It is an automatic process. We don't debate in our mind whether we are going to stop at them. We just stop!

You can travel through a small town and stop at several red lights, and if I asked you thirty minutes later how many red lights you stopped at going through that last town, many times you might say, "Were there any red lights back there?" Why? Because you already had established the *habit* of stopping at red lights!

When you practice a habit long enough, it becomes automatic. We don't decide if we are going to shower, we just do it usually at the same time each day. We don't decide if we are going to brush our teeth, we just do it usually at the same time. No effort involved—we just do it!

I want you to think about the long-term enjoyment of your life. Your *self-esteem* is dependent on your *weight*.

So commit to three red lights!

TABLE II

1. No-calorie drinks
2. One helping at dinner time
3. WFOVW

If you do this, you can have what you listed in table 1

1. *Self-esteem*

2. *Clothes*

3. *Energy*

4. *Health*

5. *Etc.*

You stop at red lights so you don't end up in a wreck and get injured and hurt. You also stop so that you won't get a ticket that causes pain when you have to pay the fine.

Remember, this is not a diet. This is *changing your eating habits for the rest of your life.*

I have shown where to put up the red lights, but you have to <u>choose</u> if you will <u>erect</u> them. *Try it!* The longer you stop at them consistently, the easier it becomes until it is like taking a shower or brushing your teeth. We are ruled by our *habits,* so why not be ruled by *good* habits?

TABLE II

1. No-calorie drinks

2. One helping at meal time

3. WFOVW

(Please read out loud.)

This is a tear-out page to put in a place you can see every day.

Chapter X

SELF-ESTEEM

This is the number one reason that people want to be at a normal weight. It is defined by Webster as *confidence* and *satisfaction* in oneself.

We all want to feel good about ourselves.

Being overweight has *nothing* to do with whether you are a good or bad person. Being overweight does not make you a bad person.

Being overweight does affect your view of yourself. Therefore it affects your feeling of *happiness.* We all want to be happy, so give the three rules a try.

I think a good idea here is to get an old picture of yourself at normal weight and put it up by your daily sheet (see chapter 23), or on the tear-out sheet on the previous page.

You really need to picture yourself at where you are going. So put that picture up and realize that the time will pass, and you will get there. Three rules!

You may feel and think your weight control problem is too big of a mountain to climb. But how do you know unless you try?

There is an old Chinese expression that says, "A journey of a thousand miles starts with a single step."

You have already climbed many mountains in your life: elementary school, high school, health problems, relationship problems, raising-kids problems, jobs, building or remodeling a house, landscaping, furnishing a house, etc. These all look too big to accomplish before you start, but the time passes; and if you really try, you will succeed. Wow!

Isn't it great!

 Remember that the sun will get up tomorrow whether you follow the three rules or not.

Remember that Christmas came in the year 10, 100, 500, 1000, 1300, 1800, 1950, 1963, 1988, 2000, 2002, 2003, 2004, 2005, and guess what? It's going to come in 2006, 2010, 2015, 2025; and if you follow the *three rules*, your *self-esteem* will be great regarding your weight. You will be happier, which is what we all want.

The payback is *great*! You can do it. It is your choice to do because the adult in you is the BOSS. Don't let the child in you deceive you and *cheat* you out of your happiness. The child in you isn't bad. The child is just a child that *never* looks at the long term.

If you don't commit to the *long term,* then the adult will never be happy.

The child in you *will adapt and enjoy* the new rules after following them.

You have to decide who is going to be the BOSS. Who is going to be the BOSS? *It is your choice.*

Take control and be glad that you do have a *choice*!

Sometimes in *life,* we have a problem or a situation where we don't have a good *choice*. What if you were told by your doctor that you have a metastatic cancer and there really isn't any good treatment for it? What if you had an accident and were paralyzed from the neck down? You don't get to have a *good* choice. What if you have five children and your spouse walks out on you? You're stuck! You just have to do the best you can and realize this is going to be a long and painful road.

This is *not* the case with your weight and how you feel about yourself regarding this problem. *You do have the choice.*

Do what the adult in you knows is in your *best* interest. Don't listen to the child. Children don't *know* anything. They have to *learn* to follow the rules or they make you miserable.

Think about it? How much power does the child have? Can the child in you make you have a seizure? No. Can the child make you throw up? No. The child can tell you that you are hungry and *you* can respond by following *three simple rules.*

The sun will come up the next morning and Christmas will come on December 25.

Chapter XI

CLOTHES

Sorry, folks, at least this will be short. I am bringing it up because it is the second thing my patients are concerned about.

The only thing brought up more often or first is self-esteem.

I know I hate it when my pants are too tight. It is a hassle to go buy bigger clothes.

I guess it does make me feel bad when I have to admit I need a size 44 pants and I used to wear a size 42, 40, or 38.

Clothes are very important to a lot of people. I'm just not one of them.

Chapter XII

HEALTH

Being overweight definitely contributes to developing diabetes. It contributes to wearing out your joints and causing the pain of arthritis. It contributes to total joint replacement. It contributes to increasing your blood pressure. It contributes to heart disease. It contributes to breathing problems. It contributes to depression.

If you develop these illnesses, it costs a lot of money. It costs to pay the doctor and undergo all the tests. It costs a lot of money for the prescriptions at the pharmacy. There are side effects and possible problems anytime you take medicines. Don't get me wrong, medicines are good, and I write thousands of prescriptions; but I also see the problems that arise.

Rather than bore you with long-drawn-out scenarios on all of these, let's choose one.

Let's say you develop diabetes. You have to take one to three different medications once or twice daily. That will cost you $50-$200 a month.

Then you have to buy a glucometer machine and test your blood sugar at least daily.

You have to see the doctor at least two to three times a year. He has to refer you to an eye doctor once a year.

You then might develop problems with your kidneys, nervous system, or heart, requiring further referrals and more tests and medicine.

I didn't write this chapter to scare you. Thank goodness, we have all these specialists to manage these problems.

But wouldn't it be a lot easier to follow the three rules and save you all this agony and pain?

Chapter XIII

DIETS AND DIET PILLS

Diets don't work! That's why there are so many of them.

The only thing that works is changing your eating habits for the rest of your life.

Diet pills don't work because as soon as you stop them and return to your old eating habits, you put the weight back on.

Modified fasting programs don't work because you go back to your old eating habits. This is just a type of diet.

So this book is about the truth and the only truth about weight control for life. You may not like hearing that this is the only way to control weight for life, but at least I told you the truth.

I'm sure 75-90 percent of you already knew this. I hope this just crystallizes in your mind the truth about weight control and gives you a *simple* plan.

You can do this on your own. You may also want to see your doctor or a doctor that does give diet pills/appetite suppressants to help you get started and make it easier to follow the three rules for three to four months.

Again, the diet pills can only help. They are not the answer. The answer is changing your eating habits for the *rest of your life.*

Chapter XIV

EXCEPTIONS

1. On special days such as Thanksgiving, Christmas, birthdays and anniversaries, don't worry about rules number 2 and number 3.

2. On vacation, don't worry about rule number 2 and rule number 3.

Why? We don't want to kill the child inside of us. He/she needs to get out and play and enjoy life. What we need to do is be the boss during the other 335 days of the year. The 30 special days won't affect your weight over twenty, thirty, forty, fifty years.

These three rules have to be reasonable to live with for the rest of your life.

I figured this out because when I was on a diet many years ago, I was sad for two weeks before Thanksgiving. I give thanks for this great country we live in and all the blessings God has given me, but Thanksgiving also means time to overeat! How do you celebrate it without eating too much? So why feel sorry for yourself and suffer two weeks for one day.

I was on vacation going to Branson, Missouri, one summer and (again on a diet) noticed so many restaurant signs. I asked my beautiful wife, Denise, why there were so many signs this time.

She laughed and said, "That is because you are on a diet!" This didn't seem fair. I work all year and then go on vacation and, I can't have an ice cream at 2:00 p.m.? I go out to eat at a good restaurant and I have to worry about the portion size? So I made this exception because the plan has to be reasonable and practical in a way that you can follow the rest of your life.

Again, these days will only total up to about thirty days.

30 days/year x 30 years= 900 days

335 day/year x 30 years= 10,050 days

I have also found that I don't overeat nearly as much on these days because I'm used to eating one helping!

3. Alcohol. A drink of alcohol, which means basically a beer, a glass of wine, or a mixed drink, has about 120 calories again. So if you only drink occasionally, this won't interfere with your overall weight. If you are concerned about it, then eat a low-calorie meal that day. If you drink too much—well, that is why they call them beer bellies, and I have no answer.

Chapter XV

EXERCISE

A book about weight without talking about exercise?

Yes!

Nah, I have to talk about this.

But my premise is that 90 percent of weight control is about calories in.

Exercise is about calories out. It is good for us healthwise and can help us control our weight.

66

The problem to me (concerning weight control for the rest of your life) is that you have to walk twenty to thirty minutes to burn up the calories in one Coke! Which is easier: drinking a low-calorie drink or walking for twenty to thirty minutes? Eating a small Snickers (2.07 ounces = 280 calories) or walking for thirty to forty minutes? Eating a small bag of chips (1 ounce = 150 calories) or walking for twenty-five to thirty minutes?

I think most of us don't exercise because:

1. we don't have the time or;
2. we are too tired.

I do try to get my patients to exercise. It is good. I try to get them to walk at least one block a day. The trick is, again, establishing a habit.

If you commit to this, you will soon find one block seems like only a few steps and you will *naturally* go farther. Don't push it!

Let's say after one week you increase to two blocks. After a few weeks, this will seem like nothing, and then you will be walking three blocks.

The idea would be working up to about twenty to thirty minutes of walking daily.

The trick to do this is to remember you are only obligated to one block a day.

So if you have worked up to six blocks and one day you don't have the time or are too tired, just walk one block that day.

The trick is to smile ☺ at the end of the block and as you turn to go home, say, "I did my exercise!" Don't get down on yourself about it but realize soon you will feel like walking farther than a block. Again, the trick is to walk at least the one block every day and give yourself the time to develop the habit. Always feel good and pat yourself on the back for the one block.

It doesn't have to be walking, but I think the important thing is some kind of commitment to at least a small amount of exercise *every day* for the rest of your life, doing any kind of exercise you enjoy.

I don't want to sound negative about exercise, but I still believe *weight control is 90 percent about calories in.*

The Three Rules

1. No-Calorie Drinks

2. One Helping at Meals

3. WFOVW

Chapter XVI

THE ROLLER COASTER

Let me explain how a diet works. It is like being on a roller coaster.

When the roller coaster is at the top, it is like when you are overweight. You're unhappy with yourself. Then you decide to go on a diet and the roller coaster is going downhill. You are feeling better, but you are still suffering while you are going down to the bottom. When you get to the bottom, meaning your normal weight you now feel good. The problem with the diet is that as soon as you get to the bottom, you go back to eating the way you did before. This results in you gaining weight, meaning you are going uphill on the roller coaster and feeling unhappy with the weight gain. Then you get to the top and are really unhappy with being overweight. You stay there until you decide to go on a diet. You feel better as you are losing weight, but it is continuous effort.

Then you get back to normal weight and feel good about yourself again. But now that your diet and goal is met, you return to your old eating habits, start to gain weight (going up the roller coaster), and feel bad again about your self-image.

So now, we end up back at the top of the roller coaster and unhappy.

When you do this for twenty, thirty, forty, or fifty years and look back, you will find you were happy for maybe two to five years (at the bottom/normal weight) and unhappy for 90 percent of your time that you were at the top of the roller coaster or on the way up or down on the ride.

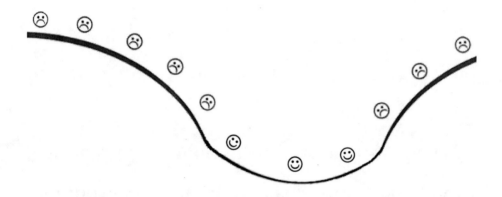

Eleven Unhappy Portions Of Time in your life compared to approximately two Happy Portions Of Time.

Try my ride!

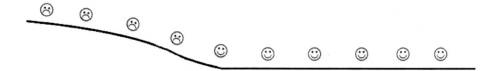

It means being relatively unhappy for a

short time while changing to being happy

for the

REST OF YOUR LIFE.

Chapter XVII

EATING OUT

This is a tough one, but let me try to help a little. You probably know more about this than I do.

Follow the three rules. Most meals at restaurants give you one and a half to two helpings.

Try doing the WFOVW before you go. Order the doggie bag when you order your food and put anything more than one helping in the doggie bag before you start eating. When you get down to the last bite, get up and go to the bathroom.

When I eat out, I often order the *large* size and put two-thirds of it in the doggie bag and have two more meals later at home. Yeah, I'm kind of cheap.

I'm sure other books have a lot of good ideas on this, but I'm keeping this simple (three rules) because I want you to have a plan that you can follow for the next twenty, thirty, forty, or fifty years.

Don't complicate things with a lot of rules. Keep it simple.

It will work!

Chapter XVIII

GOING TO PARTIES

You probably know how to handle this better than I do.

For one thing, you probably don't go to that many "coffee or tea" parties, but here are a few ideas to try to help.

Do the WFOVW before you leave to go to the event. When you get there, drink something that has no calories if possible.

If you feel you have to eat a piece of cake or eat more cookies—go ahead! I don't think this is too many calories in the long run.

If you want to make up for these extra calories, then eat a lunch that is low calorie or exercise more that day.

Chapter XIX

HOW FAST?

The speed of weight loss is not important. Changing your eating habits for the rest of your life is.

Now, I know your *brain* is mainly concerned about what those scales say! "When will I get to my goal?"

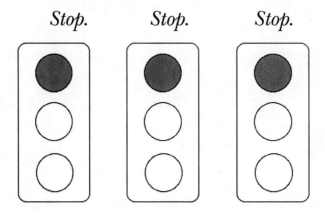

Stop.   *Stop.*   *Stop.*

The important thing is that when you arrive at your destination (goal weight), you are able to stay there for the next twenty, thirty, forty, or fifty years.

But to answer your question (how fast?), I will give you a scenario. When you decide to follow the three rules, watch what happens.

1. No-calorie drinks. If you cut one Coke/milk/ juice a day you just saved 120 calories.
2. If you only ate one helping at meals, you just cut out approximately 200-300 calories per day.
3. If you followed WFOVW between meals, you cut out at least 200-300 calories per day.

If you add up these, you are cutting out 500-800 calories a day.

500 calories/day x 30 days = 15,000 calories or about four pounds in a month

Remember, these are conservative figures. So what are you going to weigh one year from now? You should weigh 45-50 pounds less.

This whole book is to get you to see that the only thing that works is to *change your eating habits for the rest of your life.*

If you want to know what you should weigh, you can look it up on a growth chart or you can calculate it as follows:

Male—105 pounds for the first 5' + 6 pounds for every inch taller.

Therefore a male 5'8" tall should weigh 105 (for the first 5' tall) + 6 x 8 = 48 for the 8" taller than 5'. This equals 153 pounds. You then add or subtract 10 percent depending on whether you have a small frame or large frame. This gives a range of 142-168.

For a female 5'3", it is 100 pounds for the first 5' tall + 5 pounds for every inch over 5'. Therefore it would be 100 + 15 = 115 pounds, and again it is minus 10 percent for small frames (104 pounds) or plus 10 percent for large frames (126 pounds).

So let's say you are a 5'4"-female and weigh 200 and wants to weigh 130 pounds. If you start the three rules and lose 3 to 4 pounds a month, you will weigh 152 pounds after one year and will be down to your goal of 130 pounds in another six months. So it will take about a year and a half to go from 200 to 130 pounds.

But, now that you have changed your eating habits, you get to keep it off for the next 20, 30, 40, or 50 years.

You may say, "I don't want to wait a year and a half to get to my goal!" I don't blame you, but that's the way it works. I'm explaining a plan that *really* works for life.

So if you are thirty-three, and you do this for over a year and a half, then you will be thirty-four or thirty-five and get to enjoy normal weight for *forty* more years.

You can't finish high school without committing for *four* years.

You can't finish college without committing for *four* years.

You can't finish graduate school without committing to *two to four* years.

You can't raise children without committing to at *least eighteen* years.

There is no *magic* way to control your weight without changing your eating habits.

It is not how fast the weight comes off. It is all about eating habits. _You change_ your _eating habits_ and _the weight will come off and_ _stay off_!!

Chapter XX

MOMMA

Boy, was I lucky. I had a great mother who taught me a lot. I want to share two things with you.

My dad left my mother when I was nine or ten. She was a waitress and had to raise five of us kids by herself. She paid $15-a-month rent. The roof leaked, and we had one cold-water faucet on the back porch. We bathed in a washtub, and she heated the water on the stove. Our bathroom was the outhouse. But she loved us and was a good person.

One thing she used to always say when I would be going through a hard time was, "This too, my son, will pass." She didn't invent the saying, but she did teach it to me by repetition. I bring this up because if you decide to commit to the three rules, then I want you to know that the difficulty in the beginning of the action I have discussed (one helping and getting up from the table, WFOVW, and no-calorie drinks) *will also pass*—it will get easier. The payback is a great deal. It's called <u>HAPPINESS</u>!

Another great lesson she taught me is that if you try as hard as you can—you cannot fail. Wow! I was about fourteen or fifteen then.

Trying to understand this, I asked her a question, "What if I want to be the quarterback of the high school football team?"

(I'm not any better than average as an athlete. I was probably five feet seven inches and 120 pounds.)

I'm thinking this will disprove her statement. So Mom says, "If you try as hard as you can and don't become a quarterback, then you didn't fail—you just found out that you're not a quarterback."

Fear of failure prevents us from even trying to do what we want to do.

I was afraid of passing in the Nuclear Power School in the Navy.

I was afraid of going to the University of Oklahoma for my undergraduate work.

I was afraid of being able to make good grades in physics, calculus, organic chemistry, and several other courses.

I was afraid I wouldn't get accepted to medical school.

I was afraid about getting married.

I was afraid about seeing my first patient on my own.

But guess what? I succeeded in all the above because I *tried*.

So please, realize that you can be happy about how you feel about yourself if you will commit and *try*!

Three simple rules.

Do not let the fear of failure keep you from trying.

You can do it—I promise, it is worth it.

Take action. Do the three rules.

Chapter XXI

AFRAID AND FEAR vs. TERRIBLE AND FRIGHTFUL

FEAR—An unpleasant, often strong *emotion* caused by anticipation or awareness of danger.

AFRAID—Filled with concern or regret over an unwanted situation.

TERRIBLE—Suggests painfulness to great to be endured

FRIGHTFUL—Implies a startling or outrageous quality that induces utter consternation or *paralysis* from fear.

Four strong words. Having fear and being afraid are unavoidable. I'm sure you will experience these as you consider whether to start the journey of three rules.

But please don't buy into thinking this change is *terrible* or *frightful*. Reread the definition. Terrible means *pain* too great; *frightful* implies *paralysis* from *fear*. Think about the difference!

I'm not asking you to try something *terrible* or *frightful*!

The three rules are somewhat fearful, but the longer you decide to follow them, then the easier they become; and the feeling of fear turns to the feeling of success.

Someone who quits smoking goes through exactly the same thing. But all those that do quit are happy and proud of themselves for doing it. If it didn't get easier the longer you quit, then no one would quit!

The same analogy can be said to the alcoholic. Don't you know that they are fearful and afraid when they "jump on the wagon?" But if they think it's going to be terrible (painfulness too great to be endured) or *frightful* (paralysis from fear), they can't quit drinking.

These three rules will work for most but not for those who have deep psychological problems such as severe depression that is untreated. This book doesn't address anorexia nervosa or bulimia. This book is for the 90 percent that want a way to control their weight so they can feel good about themselves. Changing your eating habits is the only thing that works.

Life offers opportunities—a person just has to step out and take advantage of them.

The child in us tries to fool us by telling us that something is too hard or painful. The child tries to make us afraid and think that it would be terrible to change.

"Don't try out to be a cheerleader."

"Don't try to make the baseball team."

"Don't try to finish high school."

"Don't try college."

"Don't try marriage and kids."

"Don't try for the better job" etc. ad nauseam.

It is the child that is scared. I was scared of the *dark* until I was twenty-four and used to keep a light on at night. I didn't like myself for being afraid. So one night, I just turned it off and said out loud, "Boogeyman, if you're out there, you're just going to have to get me!" Ha-ha. I was right—there wasn't a boogeyman out there, and so I didn't have to worry about the dark the past thirty years. The child got used to the dark and quit bothering me.

We have the opportunity to listen to the adult in us and choose to let the adult be the boss and get good things in life, or we can choose to let the child in us be the boss and be unhappy.

Thank God we have a choice!

Chapter XXII

HOW AM I DOING?

We all want to see how we are doing when we start an adventure. School has grades. The boss has a paycheck. A diet has scales.

I want to reiterate that the problem is your bad habits. So rather than weigh on scales, I want you to set up a big box calendar and draw three red lights on every date. Actually, I have included this in the next twelve pages for you to use.

Each morning when you read the daily page (it only takes 30 seconds!) I want you to also color each *O* on the red light which REPRESENTS the three rules you stopped at yesterday. If you can color all 3 circles in the red lights, you made a perfect score. You are establishing eating habits for the *rest of your life.* The weight will come off and, *most* importantly, stay off.

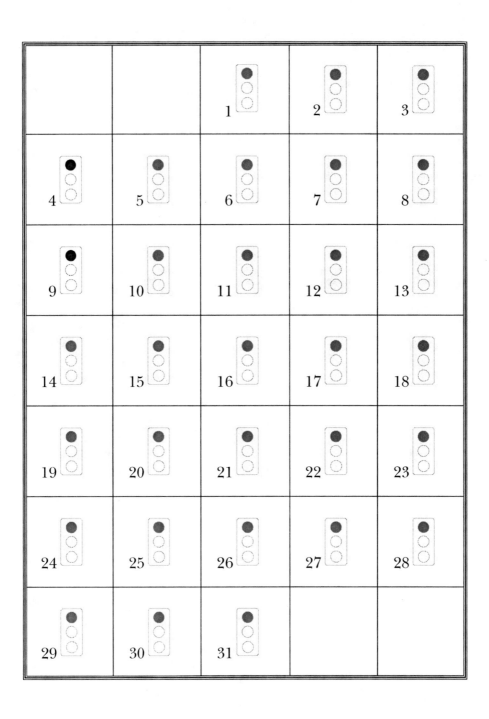

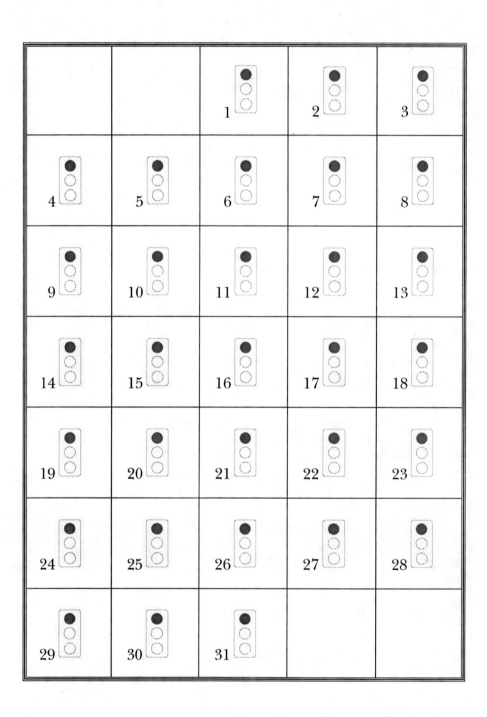

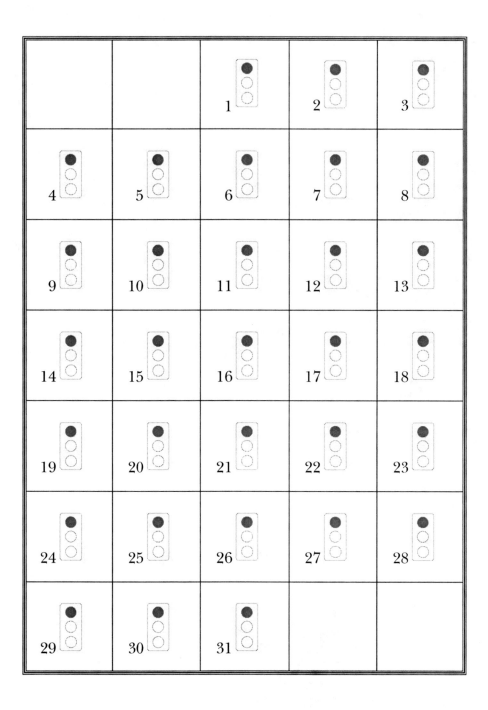

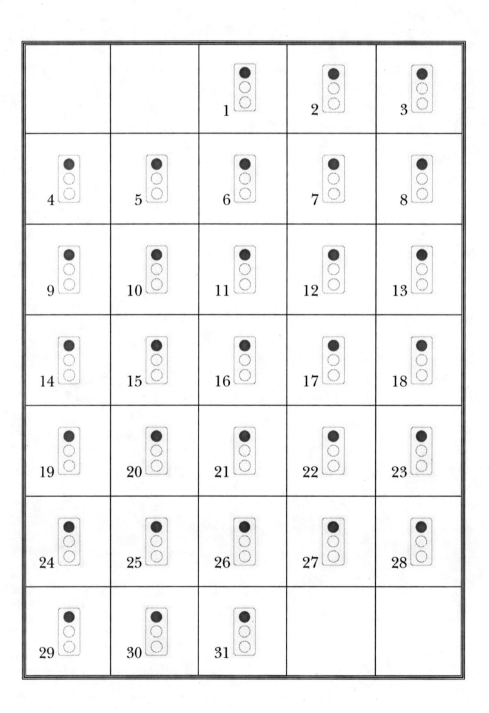

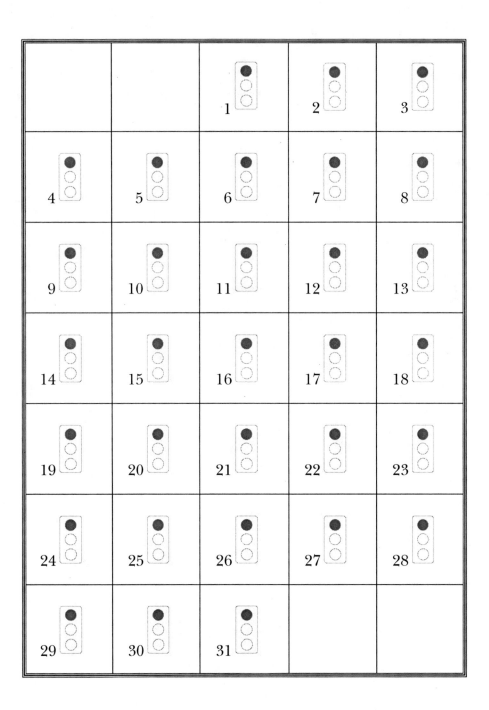

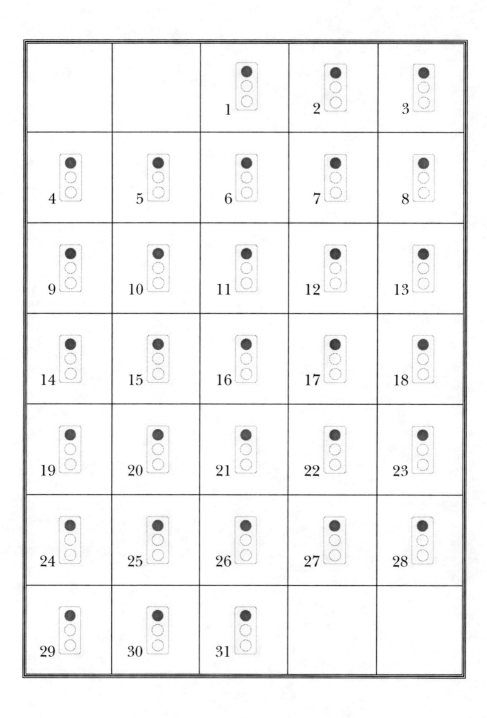

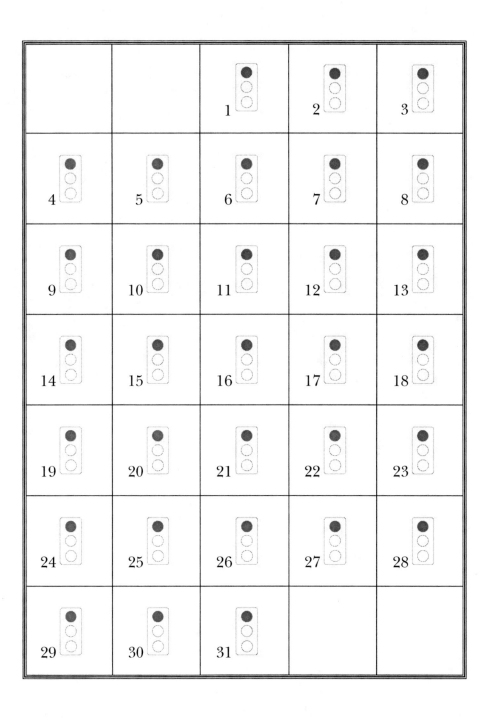

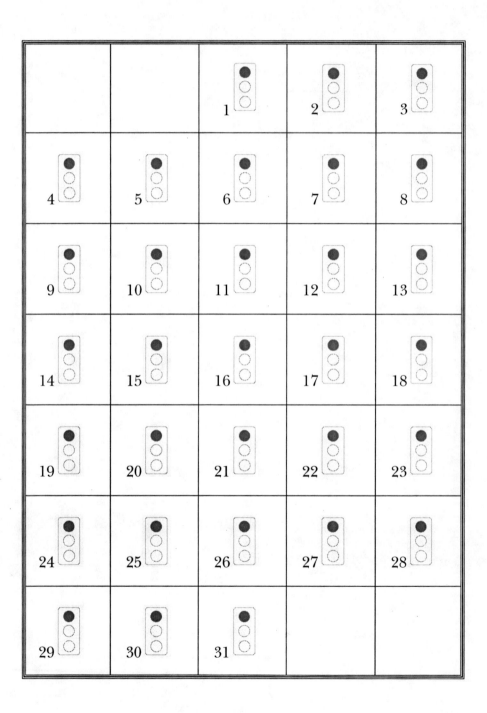

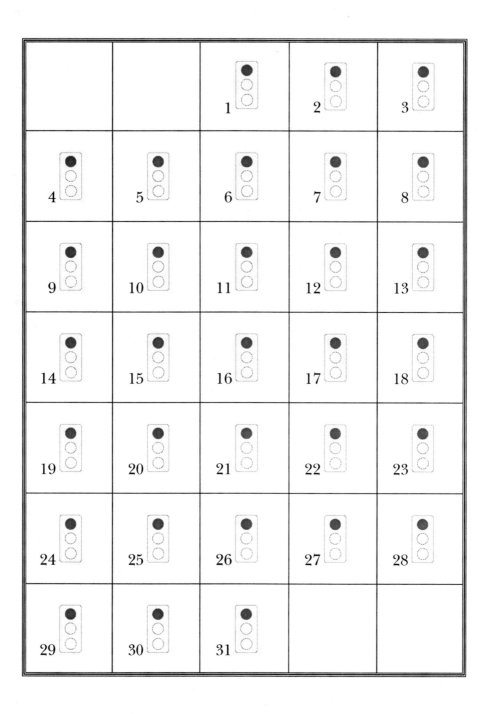

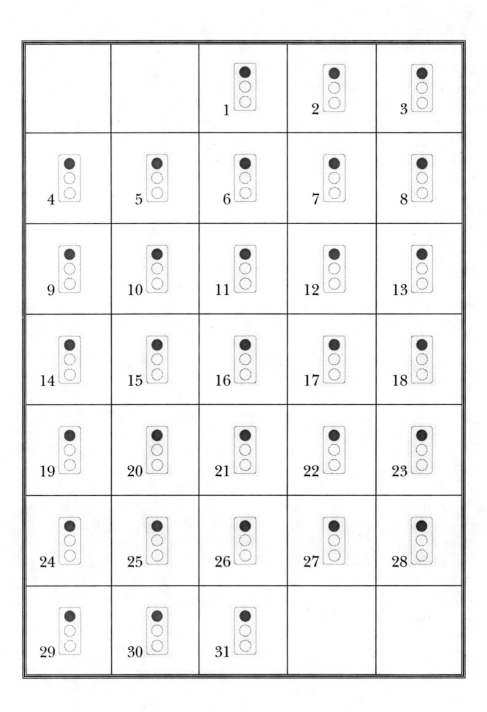

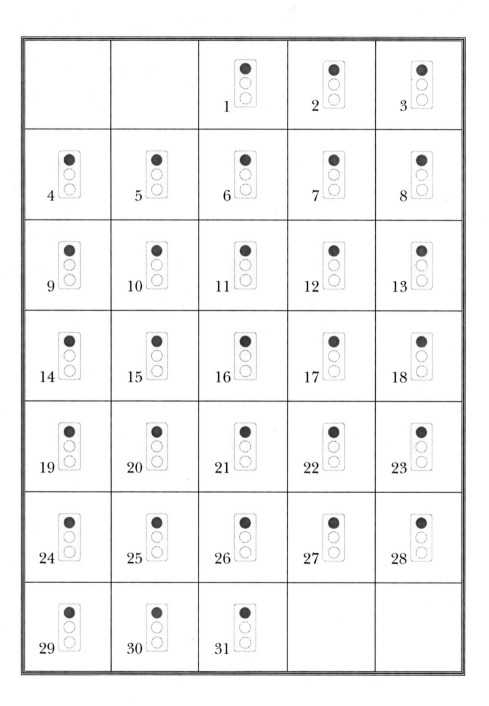

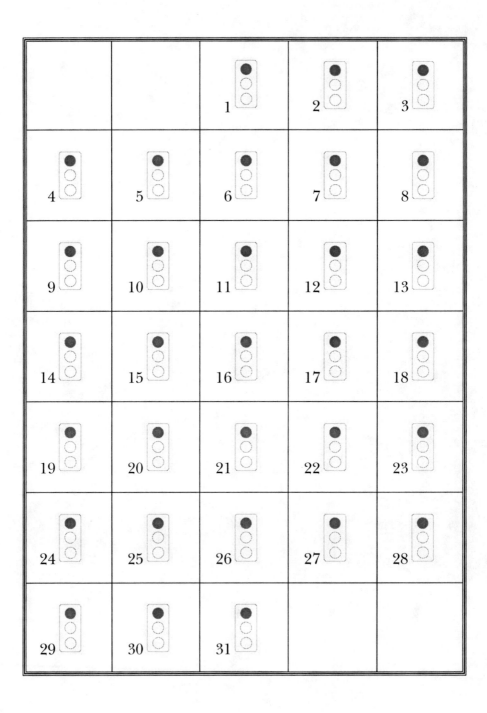

Chapter XXIII

THE DAILY PAGE

I recommend you use this next page or make your own page to read every day.

I recommend you put it on your refrigerator or bathroom mirror. It would also be good to put another one in your car or at work.

Read it daily. It only takes about thirty seconds to read the following six steps.

You need to read it *every day,* so that you *know* why and what to do. Every day for only thirty seconds, *Read it out loud.*

Copy the things you listed on page 21.

1._____

2._____

3._____

4._____

5._____

6._____

7._____

8._____

1. What's in it for me? I get the things in the box above.

2. I will get *hungry.*

3. I will *look* at my *watch.*

4. If it is mealtime, I will eat *one* helping.

5. If it is *between meals,* I will *act* and do *WFOVW.*

6. *No-calorie drinks!*

You should now have three things in line.

1. Picture of yourself
   at your goal weight.
   ☺

2. The Daily Page
   This is page 108

3. Your calendar with
   the red lights
   provided.

Doing these three things will take you only thirty seconds in the morning.

Chapter XXIV

CONGRATULATIONS—
NOW WHAT?

Congratulations! Now that you have met your goal (yea!), what do we do?

By following the three rules you have been losing weight, and now we have to talk about changes that we can make to maintain that weight for the rest of your life.

We don't need to lose any more weight so you can take in more calories and maintain your weight.

Remember calories (equals weight) come into the body in only one of these three ways:

1. At meals
2. Between meals
3. Drinks

This is where you have to be honest with yourself about where and what you are going to change. You are going to have to think and individualize your strategy and form a plan.

I'll give you some ideas, but remember, each of you is different and need to work on making some small changes. It may take trying some different things to make it work. Therefore here are some ideas that I think are good points to start with.

1. Don't mess with the no-calorie drinks.

        Exception: If you were one of those that
        gave up a glass of juice or milk once a
        day for breakfast, you can probably go
        back to drinking that one glass of juice or
        milk. Definitely, don't go back to Cokes
        or adding regular sugar to drinks.

2. Don't mess with one helping of food at meals.
    For the rest of your life, continue to practice
    one helping of food at meals.

3. This is where I have an idea that will work for
    some and not for others. Before you try it,
    be sure and make up your mind that you will
    change your plan if you can't do this and if
    you are gaining weight.

I like the idea of making a rule that once a day, you can have a snack of whatever you want. For instance, let's say you are planning or going to the movies on a Friday night and know that you will be having popcorn. Knowing your snack for the day is going to be at the movies, that means no cake with lunch or pie after dinner or midafternoon snack. If you can discipline yourself to one snack a day, your weight will stay stable at your goal weight that you have achieved.

On the other hand, if you are like some people and once you start snacking you can't stop, this change isn't for you. You will have to work something else out.

My advice is to monitor your weight once weekly on scales. If you have gained three pounds over your goal weight then you are going to have to change the plan you developed after reaching your goal. Remember, the overall basis of three simple rules are for life.

If you have a sweet tooth, you might try something I do. I carry a low calorie hard candy like low-calorie (six) LifeSavers, Sweet'N Low, Crystal Light Sugar Free with (six) calories, or many others like these. You can eat fifteen to twenty of these throughout the day and not gain weight because the total calories is fewer than in one Coke or one-half of a Snickers bar. Sucking on one low-calorie hard candy (six calories) even lasts longer—maybe four to five times as long as you would eat half of a Snickers bar.

You know, having written this, it is probably a good idea to use these hard, low-calorie candies when you start the program to lose weight!

To sum it up, *congratulations*, for changing your eating habits and reaching *your goal*. Like most things we accomplish in life, a lot of you are looking backward and thinking, "You know, it really wasn't that hard, and I am so happy being at my goal weight."

Finally, remember this is *not* a diet you have been on. This is a decision by you to change your eating habits for the rest of your life. Three simple, reasonable rules to change your life. The real truth about being at normal weight for life!

I started to say, "Good luck," but this book has nothing to do with luck. It is about *you* making the *decision* to *change* the way *you* eat. You can do it! Make the *decision*!

Keep forming the three habits. Remember that they get easier and easier and easier and easier the longer you do them until finally it takes no effort and is just the way you do things.

Chapter XXV

CHAPTER FOR CHRISTIANS

If you are a Christian, then spending time with God in his word, and praying will also help and strengthen you. God's love is perfect, and he loves all of his children no matter what, but I also believe he wants us to be happy with ourselves and is truly interested in everyone of us. Ask *out loud* (tired of hearing me say that?) for the Holy Spirit to live in you and give you joy as you go through this adventure of *change.*

Some of my favorite verses are:

1. Greater is he that is in us than he that is in the world.

2. Cast all your cares upon Jesus, for he cares for you.

3. Ask, and you will be given. Seek, and you will find. Knock and the door will be opened. Ask God for help in changing and he will help you.

4. So don't be anxious about tomorrow. God will take care of your tomorrow too. Live one day at a time.

5. For my yoke is easy, and my burden is light.

6. I can do all things through CHRIST who strengthens me.

Here are some other Bible verses that will help you to change and have control of your weight for life. I know reading these will give you strength, peace of mind, courage, joy, and power to follow the three rules!

May I suggest you read and underline your favorite ones to read on occasions because I know I have probably listed too many! But guess what? There were so many more I wanted to include!

1.) Thou will keep him in perfect peace; because he trusteth in thee (Isa. 26:3).

2.) The Lord my God holds my right hand; he is the Lord, who says to me, "Fear not, I will help you." (Isa. 41:13).

3.) Oh that men would praise the Lord for his goodness, and for his wonderful works to the children of men for he satisfieth the longing soul and filleth the hungry soul with goodness (Pss. 107: 8-9).

4.)   I beseech you therefore, brethren, by the mercies of God, that you present your bodies a living sacrifice, Holy, acceptable unto God, which is your reasonable service (Rom. 12:1).

5.)   Trust in the Lord with all thine heart; and lean not unto thy own understanding. In all thy ways acknowledge him, and he shall direct thy paths (Prov. 3:5-6).

6.)   He hath showed thee man, what is good; and what doth the Lord require of thee, but to do justly, and to love mercy, and to walk humbly with thy God (Mic. 6:8).

       (This probably doesn't relate to helping you follow the three rules, but it is my favorite verse in the Old Testament. I just wanted to share it with you.)

7.)   If God be for me, who can be against me? (Rom. 8:31)

8.)   He that hath no rule over his own spirit is like a city that is broken down without walls (Prov. 25:28).

9.)   Better is the end of a thing than a beginning of thereof; and the patient in Spirit is better than the proud in Spirit. (Eccles. 7:8).

10.)   For God hath not given us the spirit of fear; but of power, and of love, and of a sound mind (2 Tim. 1:7).

11.)   It is God's desire that I be free from all anxiety and distressing care (1 Cor. 7: 32).

12.)   And when he was at the place Jesus said unto them pray that ye enter not into temptation (Luke 22:40).

13.) The boundary lines have fallen from me in pleasant places; surely I have his life full inheritance. (Ps. 16:6) (The three rules can be your boundary line.)

14.) And Jesus said unto them, I am the bread of life; He that cometh to me, shall never hunger; And he that believeth on me shall never thirst (John 6:35).

15.) But I see another law in my members warring against the law of my mind and bringing me into captivity to the law of sin which is in my members. Oh wretched man that I am! Who shall deliver me from the body of this death? I thank God, through Jesus Christ our Lord. So then, with the mind I myself serve the law of God; but with the flesh the law of sin (Rom. 7: 23-25).

16.) So shall my word be that goeth forth out of my mouth; it shall not return unto me void, but it shall accomplish that which I please, and it shall prosper in the thing whereto I sent it (Isa. 55: 11).

17.) Rejoicing in hope; Patient and tribulation; Continuing instant in prayer (Rom. 12:12).

18.) My brethren, count all joy when you fall into diverse temptations; knowing this, that the trying of your faith worketh patience. But let patience have her perfect work that yee may be perfect and entire wanting of nothing. (James 1:2-4) (I'm not happy when the way is rough but I have always been happy after going through a rough time and either changed a bad habit or just done the right thing.)

19.) And he said unto me, my grace is sufficient for thee; for my strength is made perfect in weakness. Most gladly therefore will I rather glory in my infirmities, that the power of Christ may rest upon me (2 Cor. 12:9).

20.) Lord, my heart is not hearty, nor my eyes lofty, neither do I exercise myself in great matters or in things to high for me. Surely I have behaved in quieted myself as a child that is weaned of his mother my soul is even as a weaned child (Pss. 131:1-2).

21.) For by wise council thou shall make thy war and in multitude of counts there, there is safety (Prv 24:6). (I think this is a place that joining weight watchers or Tops can help you. Groups with the same problem draw strength and encouragement, peace and success from each other.)

22.) That I rejoiced in the Lord greatly, that now at the last your care of me have flourished again; wherein you were also careful, but you lacked opportunity. Not that I speak in respect of want; for I have learned, in what so ever state I'm in there with be content (Phil 4:10-11).

23.) I can do all things through Christ, which strengthen me (Phil 4:13).

24.) And he spake a parable unto them to this end, that men are always to pray and not to faint, quit or to give up (Luke 18:1).

25.) For I know the thoughts that I think towards you, saith the Lord, thoughts of peace, and not of evil, to give you an expected end (Jer. 29:11).

26.) For the word of God is quick, and powerful, and sharper than any two edge sword, piercing even to the dividing of sunder and soul and spirit, and of the joints and marrow, and is a discerner of the thoughts of the intents of the heart (Heb. 4:12).

27.) God wants me to prosper and be in health, even as my soul prosper (3 John 1:2).

28.) But they that wait upon the Lord shall renew there strength; they shall mount up with wings as eagles; they shall run, and not be weary, and they shall walk, and not faint (Isa. 40:31).

29.) I trusted in, relied on, and was confident in you oh Lord; I said, you are my God. My times are in your hands (Pss. 31:14-15).

30.)   And I will give unto thee the keys of the kingdom of heaven and what so ever should bind on earth shall, be bound in heaven; and what so ever shall loose on earth, shall be loosed in heaven (Matt. 16:19). (You can bind the three rules as part of your life, Christ has given you the power.)

31.)   And this is the confidence that we have in him, that if we ask anything according to his will he hearth us (1 John 5:14).

32.)   As I think in my heart, so am I (Prov. 23:7).

33.)   But my God shall supply all your need according to his riches in glory by Christ Jesus (Phil. 4:19).

34.)   All things are lawful unto me, but all things are not expedient; all things are lawful for me, but I will not be brought under the power of any (1 Cor. 6:12). (Uncontrollable eating is not helpful to you—try the three rules.)

35.) Be careful for nothing; but in everything by prayer and supplication with thanks giving let your request be made known unto God (Phil. 4:6).

36.) Have not I commanded thee? Be strong and of good courage; be not afraid, neither be though dismayed; for the Lord thy God is with thee whether so ever though goest (Josh. 1:9).

37.) And let us not be weary in well doing; for in due season we shall reap if we faint not (Gal. 6:9).

38.) Fear thou not; for I am with thee: be not dismayed; for I am thy God: I will strengthen thee; yea, I will help thee; yea, I will uphold thee with the right hand of my righteousness (Isa. 41:10).

39.) Oh that men would praise the Lord for his goodness, and for his wonderful works to the children of men! For he satisfied the longing in my soul and fill up the hungry soul with goodness (Pss. 107:8-9).

40.) Now the Lord of peace himself give you peace always by all means the Lord be with you all (2 Thess. 3:16).

41.) And he said unto me, my grace is sufficient for thee; for my strength is made perfect in weakness (2 Cor. 12:9).

42.) I am living the life of the spirit because the Holy Spirit dwells within me (Rom. 8:9).

43.) Meats for the belly, and the belly for meats; but God shall destroy both it and them. Our body is not for fornication, but for the Lord and the Lord for the body (1 Cor. 6:13).

44.) Ask and it shall be given you; seek, and you shall find; knock, and it shall be opened unto you: for everyone asketh, receiveth; and he that seeketh findeth; and to him that knocketh, it shall be opened (Matt. 7:7-8). (This is the verse I believed opened my eyes to the Lord. I think it can also be used to help us conquer a problem in our lives.)

45.) Cast thy burden upon the Lord and he shall sustain thee; he shall never suffer righteous to be moved (Ps. 55:22).

46.) That the God of our Lord Jesus Christ, the Father of glory, may give unto you the spirit of wisdom and revelation in the knowledge of him. The eyes of your understanding being enlightened; that ye may know what is the hope of his calling, and what the riches of the glory of his inheritance in the saints, and what is the exceeding greatness of his power to us—ward who believe, according to the working of his mighty power (Eph. 1:17-19).

47.)   The humble shall see this, and be glad: and your heart shall live that see God (Ps. 69:32).

The Lord is my shepherd; I shall not want. He maketh me to lie down in green pastures: he leadeth me beside the still waters. He restoreth my soul: he leadeth me in the paths of righteousness for his name's sake. Yea, though I walk through the valley of the shadow of death, I will fear no evil: for thou art with me; thy rod and thy staff they comfort me. Thou preparest a table before me in the presence of mine enemies: thou anointest my head with oil; my cup runneth over. Surely goodness and mercy shall follow me all the days of my life: and I will dwell in the house of the Lord for ever (Pss. 23:1-6)

Our father which art in heaven, Hallowed be thy name. Thy kingdom come. Thy will be done, in earth as it is in heaven. Give us this day our daily bread. And forgive us our debts, as we forgive our debtors. And lead us not into temptation, but deliver us from evil: For thine is the kingdom, and the power, and the glory forever. Amen. (Matt. 6:9-13)

My brothers and sisters in Christ, be wise and use your relationship with Christ to help you. He is waiting and *desires* your conversation and life. We are his children, he is our Father. He is a personable God.

May I make a practical suggestion to you based on what I heard from a preacher on the radio one day?

Do you have a clock? He challenged us, believers, to set our alarm clock in the morning for just five minutes earlier than we usually do and spend it with Jesus. Five minutes! I took his advise and it has made a big difference in my life. You might try reading one chapter of Proverbs (there are thirty-one, therefore read the one that corresponds to the day when you are reading), read one chapter of Psalms or read a few verses of one of the Gospels. This will only take three minutes and then spend time talking to God for one to two minutes. Just talk like in a normal conversation. Don't try to talk like "church talk."

Five minutes? Sounds easy to me. Will you do it? Will you at least try? Come on, let's do it. Ring. Ring. Ring. Five minutes!

One last idea is to sing, hum, or whistle familiar Christian songs when tempted. It is amazing how it takes your mind off what you don't want to do. There is power in the blood, and that power can easily be brought up by praising Jesus through songs.

The songs *are already in your head.* They have played hundreds and thousands of times in your mind. "Jesus Loves Me," "Trust and Obey," "Blessed Assurance," "When The Roll Is Called Up Yonder," the "Hallelujah" chorus of Handel's *Messiah,* "Amazing Grace," and "How Great Thou Art."

I dare you, when tempted, to break your rules, to sing, or hum one of these. I dare you because I want you to win and to be happy, and I know this will work.

Fight the good fight, triumph over this problem you have.

Anyone can carry his burden, however hard, until nightfall. Anyone can do his work, however hard, for one day. Anyone can live sweetly, patiently, lovingly, purely, till the sun goes down.

Sincerely, In Christ's Love and Power

Rod Linzman

Chapter XXVI

MY VIEW OF LIFE

This has nothing to do with the purpose of this book, *Weight Control for Life.* So if you are not interested, don't read it. This is a simply put story about my belief in life.

Again, this has nothing to do with the purpose of this book. Nothing to do with weight control.

I am writing this just because I want to. I had no idea I would be writing this until now when I have finished my book.

God, who is Holy (perfect, righteous and without sin), created the earth and all the life on it. He created the first two humans, Adam and Eve, and they were perfect without sin. They walked and talked with God in a perfect relationship

Then Adam and Eve were tricked by Satan (the angel one who rebelled against God and was thrown out of heaven) to sin, and God could not be in their presence anymore because God is holy.

Sin just means doing anything or thinking anything wrong. Some have explained it as missing the target of being perfect.

This did not stop God's love for all of us, but Adam and Eve's sin was passed on to all of us.

God had a plan to make us right with him again, and that was to send his only begotten son, Jesus Christ. He lived for thirty-three years and never sinned although he was tempted in all the temptations common to man. He taught us what God is like.

He was crucified and shed his blood to take on all of our sins. He was raised from the dead three days after the crucifixion and was seen by hundreds and interacted with many for about forty days before he returned to heaven.

> For God so loved the world that he gave his only begotten son that whosoever believeth in him should not perish but have eternal life (John 3:16).

Jesus, being perfect, paid for the sin Adam did and that we inherited from him. Now we can be saved from our sin. "All have sinned and come short of the Glory of God" (Rom. 3:23).

May I suggest you read the book of Mark to get to know more about who Jesus is and what he taught.

It is as simple as believing this historical account and believing in Jesus. You just have to acknowledge you are a sinner and pray for him to forgive you and invite him into your life to be Savior and Lord. He will do the rest. You can do it right now—you need no one else. The Holy Spirit will guide you.

Here are the *ABCs* of Salvation.

Admit you have sinned (Ps. 32:5). God loves everyone and wants all to become members of his family, but sin keeps us apart from God (Isa. 59:2). The Bible says all have sinned (Rom. 3:23).

Believe Jesus is God's Son. He took the punishment for your sins on himself by dying on the cross (Rom. 5:8). You must believe that he is God and that he died to offer you forgiveness (Acts 10:43).

Confess your sins (1 John 1:8-9) You must
be truly sorry for your sins, forsake them,
and ask Jesus to forgive you (Acts 3:19).

If you want to talk to someone about it, go to a Bible-believing church, and there are plenty of people who would love to talk to you about it.

There are many, many questions, whys, ifs, and other things to talk about and argue about, but the above story is all that is really important.

Some people don't come to Jesus because they don't want someone to run their life. Some are "intellectuals" who think all of life evolved. Some people believe, by living a good life, it will make them right with God. Some people think that God is a kill joy that just doesn't want us to have fun.

There are many other reasons people use not to accept Jesus. You know what is really neat about God? He is *love*. Think about it—you can't have *love* unless you have a *choice*. God *will not force* you to believe in him and the historical facts about his son, Jesus. He loves you so much he gives that *choice* to you. God states he hopes none will perish but that all would be saved through belief and acceptance of Christ.

My prayer is that you would choose to accept Jesus who took on our sins so that he may be your Savior. Being saved and being made right with God is the most important thing in life. It is a decision for eternity. God loves you and wants to be your perfect loving Father.

Sincerely, In Christ Love,

Rod

This book is dedicated to the Glory of God

100 SHOUT WITH JOY before the Lord, O earth! [2] Obey him gladly; come before him, singing with joy.

[3] Try to realize what this means—the Lord is God! He made us—we are his people, the sheep of his pasture.

[4] Go through his open gates with great thanksgiving; enter his courts with praise. Give thanks to him and bless his name. [5] For the Lord is always good. He is always loving and kind, and his faithfulness goes on and on to each succeeding generation.

Postscript

I started writing this book so that I could save time from explaining all this to each patient who came to see me to lose weight. I just didn't have time to tell them the *truth* about how to control their weight by changing their eating habits.

As a family doctor I take care of everything, i.e., diabetes, hypertension, emphysema, pediatrics, heart failure, angina, infections, dermatology, pneumonia, stomach ulcer disease, gallbladder disease, broken bones, and mainly every kind of problem you can imagine. I have worked covering the emergency room for twenty-five years. These are the things I do most of the time. Weight problems are a small part of my practice, and I wrote the book so people can understand their problem and have a plan that is simple and reasonable to treat them more thoroughly. The key word in this book is *change*. Now that I have written it, I realize that that is the key to solving any problems we have. If you do drugs, you have to *change*. If you drink too much alcohol, you must *change*. If you have been put in *prison* for doing something wrong, you must change.

There is no room here for feeling sorry for yourself because we all have at least some kind of problem we need to *change* for the rest of our life. We are all in the same *boat*.

I don't think I brought up the fact that as you start on this adventure that many of you will "fall off the wagon" at one time or another.

When you go to fill in the circles on the red light and have to admit you will have a feeling of failure. The truth is you did fail yesterday in some way of following the rules. So what should you do?

1) The worst thing to do is feel bad or guilty about yourself.

2) The *best* thing you can do is *admit* it and simply say, "I will follow the rules today."

Remember, it is the tortoise that wins the race. It is the person who gets up when knocked down that finally wins the fight. It isn't the smartest or the strongest that wins as often as the person who keeps their eyes on the target and "keeps on keeping on."

There are thousands of examples of how *persistence* wins out over other qualities.

You need to talk out loud about your positive accomplishments. Say out loud, "Yes!" when you Color In a circle on the red light for no-calorie drink. Say out loud, "Yes!" when you limit yourself to one helping at meals. Say, "Yea!" out loud when you did WFOVW in between meals.

You have to read the daily sheet *daily* out loud and renew your brain with all the *good* things you get for *changing*.

Smile, be happy about it.

Be careful of other people and their advice and of a million different ways of losing weight and dieting. Remember, this is your deal. I guarantee it will work.

You must believe (because it is the truth) that the longer you follow these rules, the easier it will become. I promise. You have to see the vision of the long term in you mind's eye; see it?

I am not opposed to and actually believe that weight watchers or similar programs are good. Incorporate all their ideas and support into this program. They can teach you many things that will help and not make you break your three rules.

Biography

Dr. Rod Linzman is a fifty-seven-year-old family physician, practicing for the past twenty-five years in the small southern Oklahoma towns of Madill for ten years and Waurika for fifteen years.

Ninety percent of his medical practice is mainly in-house care of hospital patients, ER treatment, and clinic practice, averaging approximately sixty hours a week. He delivered babies and assisted on major surgeries during his first eight to ten years of practice but had to give that up due to malpractice liability charges and technological advances.

Approximately 90 percent of his patients is the above and 10 percent is in helping people control their weight. He did not have the time to spend two to three hours explaining what he has written in this book and therefore wrote it to save him time and possibly help thousands of people with their weight problem. He states, "Being overweight causes more health problems than heart disease."

He has been married for thirty years to his wife, Denise, who is also his best friend. He expresses his gratitude for her adapting to his profession which requires him to be gone many hours at night and hundreds of seventy-two-hour weekends in the ER.

He describes her as beautiful, wonderful, strong, fun, and having the greatest smile. He prayed for a wife and believes God gave her to him.

Dr. Linzman is most thankful for being led to Christ as a thirteen-year-old boy at First Baptist

Church in Hugo, Oklahoma, where he grew up and graduated from high school in 1968.

With the Vietnam War going on and the draft in place, he chose to join the USN where he committed six years and was trained to operate nuclear power plants.

He then served six years and helped operate the nuclear reactors aboard the nuclear-powered carrier *Enterprise*. He made two nine-month tours to Vietnam, received a commendation, and was honorably discharged in December 1974.

Dr. Linzman states God had led him to attempt to be a "country family doctor," and after undergraduate studies at the University of Oklahoma, he was accepted and graduated from Oklahoma State University College of Osteopathic Medicine and Surgery in 1981.

He and Denise have two sons, Dan and Gib, who are married to two wonderful young ladies, Jamie and Andi. They have been blessed with two miracles—their grandchildren, Ainsley and Cole. He states they all are his most important things in life, and he is very proud of them.

Printed in the United States
142320LV00003B/27/P